Footprin   n

Eileen M Taylor

chipmunkapublishing
the mental health publisher

All rights reserved, no part of this publication may be reproduced by any means, electronic, mechanical photocopying, documentary, film or in any other format without prior written permission of the publisher.

>Published by
>Chipmunkapublishing
>United Kingdom

http://www.chipmunkapublishing.com

Copyright © Eileen M Taylor 2014

ISBN   978-1-78382-082-5

Chipmunkapublishing gratefully acknowledge the support of Arts Council England.

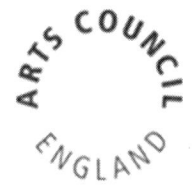

'Though leaves are many, the root is one;

Through all the lying days of my youth

I swayed my leaves and flowers in the sun;

Now I may wither into the truth.'

The Coming of Wisdom with Time

W. B. Yeats

Eileen M Taylor

Footprints On The Moon

The air is still. Still what? Still here? Yes, although it is hard to see. Haze on the horizon makes the world seem smaller, the edge closer. Perhaps it is. Today I am standing on a beach in the sun and breathing the still air. It is not a usual day. It is warm, for a start. Hot even. I can feel my shoulders burning and begin to worry about skin cancer. My head throbs in the heat and fills up with tumours in my mind, which is elsewhere. The beach is deserted, a strange way to describe an expanse of sand. In any case, it is empty of people at least. Except me. I am looking out to sea. To see what? Who knows? So much constant liquid shifting, such impermanence. It all seems very appealing. No traces left, no clues. I am not in hiding; I just don't want to be found. There is a difference. I can still hear her voice, so shrill, accusing, and hurt. But that was a long time ago. Surely all that should be gone by now. Time heals, isn't that what they say? Things fade in time. Memories though… they are not in time, they are in our heads. What makes them fade? If we can control what is in our minds then it is only logical that we can rid ourselves of unwanted memories. If not, then we cannot even choose what gets in there in the first place and there is nothing we can do. Free will and determinism. An age old problem. There is never going to be an answer so why even consider the question (unless, of course, it has been determined that we will)? So many complications to make an already difficult situation even more problematic. Being is a tricky business. Today the sky is intense. Heated and blue. No clouds. Clear view of the star that is the centre of the universe (according to us, at least). A universe that is constantly expanding. I can't understand that at all. A universe is, by definition, universal. Infinite. So where is it expanding to? Into what? What is beyond infinity, and how can that be? My small mind is boggling, and even more so when it considers that the word boggle actually exists and means something. Still. The sand is hot between my toes and I am far enough up the beach to avoid the slight displacement of air the tide washes in. Soon the sun will slip silently down towards the furthest point of my vision. (A more comfortable thought than that where I am standing is tipping up backwards at hundreds of miles an hour. Always bending truths to find the easiest to accept.) Darkness is waiting in the wings to seep in and perhaps here, away from the glare of humanity, I will see the stars. The further stars. The planets. Bits of crushed rock the size of planets accelerating towards destruction. Millions of years old shiftings. Or maybe the clouds will come in and I will only see them. It is all so unpredictable. Whatever. At some point, I will have to return. Frail flesh. I have needs. Stupid, selfish and small, but needs nonetheless; food, fresh water, shelter, hygienic toilet facilities. Hell, I even need other people, although I hate to admit it. I tried not to, tried the total isolation thing for a while, no speech, no physical or mental contact of any kind. I went a little crazy. However, after just a few months of intensive psychiatric assistance, I was no longer considered subversive (my version) or a danger to myself (their's). I was once again the small, stupid, selfish and needy person I had been trying not to be. Restored. The balance redressed. Fitting in, that is what it is all about. Like those toys for the kids we all still wish we were. The square peg goes in the square hole. You are this shape and the space you live in is moulded accordingly. But don't attempt to alter your shape, you won't fit into your space any more and no good can come of it. It's uncomfortable. Others will be forced to take it upon themselves to reshape you, make you see the folly of trying to change. You cannot alter the way things are, the way things must be. Jeez and all I wanted was a different favourite colour. Anyway there are a few stars now. A sliver of moon. Clouds rolling in from where the noise of the sea is. The breeze has begun. It is time to go.

The pub is busy, smoky, and full of noise and flashing lights. Shouts and bass beats. Laughter. Electronic tunes and lights from the machines you cannot win on but play anyway – assuming, as ever, a certain swagger and the gambler's eternal faith that one day just maybe... I buy my pint and stand in the corner. My need for other people has not yet reached crisis point. The grubby lino flooring is patterned with burns, spills and cigarette ends. The tables all wobble. The wooden benches (rescued from churches in a strangely satisfying ideological shift) are hard and uncomfortable. The drinks are too expensive. Yet it is always busy. Almost every night you have to fight for each garishly covered stool, each inch of elbow room. On the next street, there is a pub with comfortable chairs and no patrons. I cannot explain it – just follow the crowds. Independent thought? That's simply not where it's at. I finish my drink and go. I have an early start. Tomorrow I return to exorcise my ghost.

She's not here. Not yet. But, she will be, I'm almost certain. It's me who's been gone.

Lee and I sat in the churchyard behind the pub with a bottle of vodka. I told her my story and she held me. We cried.

The sky began to lighten. Lee still held me.

    'So where are you staying?' she asked. So strong and practical.

'I just got here. Nothing with me. Didn't know how welcome I'd be. Have to go back in two days. Gotta keep my appointments. Thought I'd just sleep out.' I was always a little stupid that way. Spent so many drunken nights in so many unsafe places that a couple of summer nights in my old hometown didn't seem unreasonable or daunting. Lee took my hand.

'We're going to mine before the birds start singing. We can work things out there. I'm cold.'

'I'm colder. In so many ways.' I could never resist a little melodrama.

'Away with you,' she said with so much compassion that I nearly wept again. The streets were empty. Something about a city street with nobody on it – always makes me think I am the last person alive in the world, the unwitting survivor of some silent nuclear disaster. Of course, it usually just means that I've been out all night again and really it's just far too late or far too early to be wandering. Sometimes you can see the haar and the sun melting it away. But that's only on good mornings and I haven't had too many of those. I let Lee lead me through the dawn.

Her house was in Tollcross. It took us half an hour to reach it under the pink-streaked sky. She showed me in and put on the kettle. Normality, it seemed to me - houses, kettles, sofas, and power showers. Pictures on the walls. One I'd painted several years ago in better times. I thought about Beck and K as Lee made up a bed for me. My supposed friends. An admittedly substantial time away and they acted as if they did not know me, or didn't want to know me. Whichever. And it wasn't even my fault. At least not all of it was. Lee handed me a cup of tea. I think I smiled.

Sometimes when the sky clouds over I can see her face again. The way it shone so brightly, for a second, then faded into nothing. She had been the big love of my life, such as it was. We had done all the usual things. Talked of moving in together. Cats and a studio for my painting. The whole bit. She was going to carry on working to support me as I struggled on as an artist. Until I sold a few works. Got established. We both knew that was never going to happen but planned around it anyway. In fact, we both new none of it would happen. I suppose we just didn't want to face that. The ideals advancing years subdue but can never quite destroy. She was always the sensible one. The doctor. But neither of us allowed for what happens when the world interferes. We had our circle of friends. Hanging around the music scene, never giving up on the idea that we all had something to say. Something to create. Something to make our names even locally although our dreams were bigger than that. Beck, the doctor, publishing articles in various periodicals, was the most grounded, ostensibly the highest achiever. But she wanted to write crime thrillers. K was a musician on the dole waiting for her big break. Lee temped in offices during the day and took photographs by night. Her thing was people. People dressed up for theme nights and parties. People playing music. People dancing in any dodgy nightclub. We all drank a lot. Dabbled in the softer drugs and those we were prescribed for our various neuroses and depressions. Met up on Sundays for belated brunches in cafes. Hair of the dog dinners. Read the papers and talked of arty things. Or rather, derided the latest publishers, galleries, record companies that rejected us. But then I left. Left it all behind one sudden day.

Beck was at work when I got the call. I was pretty much living in my studio space at the time (our plans of co-habiting having come to little more than discussions in the pub). I did mean to leave a note but the taxi was early and I ran. Took one small bag with clean underwear and a toothbrush. Left my half-finished paintings and sculptural works-in-progress – never could stick at one thing. Thought I'd only be a couple of days. Explain it all on my return. No problem. That's what I thought. Instead... well things got a bit more complicated. The longer I stayed away, the harder it became to write or call. Nobody knew where I was and as far as my limited thinking went at the time, nobody would really care too much. After all, what was I leaving behind? A relationship and erstwhile friends, all going nowhere. Not that I was going anywhere myself. We were all just drifting. Always waiting. My brother was in trouble and he needed me. I think. Or maybe he just wanted to say goodbye. Whatever. By the morning I was gone.

Lee was at work when I woke up feeling woolly-mouthed and lonely. She'd left a note. 'Back at 5.30. Help yourself.' She could not have had any sleep at all. I opened a can of beer, lit a cigarette and switched on the TV. Wondering whether she would speak to Beck and K during what was left of the day. Especially Beck. I felt pangs of nostalgia for the way things used to be. From what Lee had told me, K now had a publishing deal for her songs and spent half of her time in London. Beck was halfway through her first novel. Where was I? Still sitting drinking. Still waiting, biding my time. In fact, I had not touched a paintbrush in almost a year. I was further from making a living from my art than I had ever been and I'd never been that close. However, none of their brothers had taken overdoses on the beach and died. None of them had taken their own overdoses and nearly died. My progress may have been a little eclipsed by events, but I did not need excuses. I had my reasons. Selfish and strange but reasons nonetheless. At least I still had Lee on my side. That was more than I had expected. Although I had not really considered expectations until I'd got to the pub the night before. Too many complications, too many... ah but what is the point of wondering? I had appointments to keep. I had things to do.

My old artwork had been kept in storage by the ever-patient landlords of the studio space. I hired a taxi and collected as much as was salvageable, took it to Lee's. She had cleared out her spare room for me. I was beginning to feel more settled. I had explained to my psychiatrists what my plans were and they had, rather charitably, agreed that any attempt to return to my old life could only be a good thing. My referral was transferred to Edinburgh and I was free from the associations of the preceding months. Or something. For the past fortnight, I'd been holed up in Lee's flat. I spent the last of my week's benefits on some canvas and paints. Thinking I'd get back to what I knew, thinking that might make a difference and things might get back to the way they had been. Fall into place. My world might begin to resolve itself into something that made sense again. I still hadn't talked to my old friends despite Lee's best efforts to alter this state of affairs. Not that they had shown any inclination to hear me out. Lee had continued to go out with the old gang but, so far, I had remained sequestered and secluded. Besides, I knew what they thought of me. Beck and K had always been close and they'd always take the same side. Even when Beck and I had been together. It was the idea of Beck hating me that was the hardest to take. We had been the golden couple on the scene. The ones everybody looked to as an example, a myth that no-one was willing to dispel. Lee had tried to talk them round but, as I'd expected, got pretty much nowhere so far. They could be stubborn when they thought they were right and even when they knew they were wrong. So what chance did I stand? I was not the same person I had been before I left and the chances were that they, too, had changed. I had more scars and a sorry tale to tell and they had got on with their lives and put me out of their minds. Now I was back.

My painting was not going well but I did not want to die anymore. One day at a time, as they say. Every day a new day to invent yourself. Every morning an opportunity to say 'hey and who to be today'. A new existential crisis for each dawn. Today I have to sort things out with Beck. That is the task – my goal. I call her. All day waiting for 6pm until she got home from work. Chewing fingernails, smoking too much and all day waiting. She answers. I say hello. She does not hang up. Not right away. Good sign number one. I tell her James died. She says 'I know, Lee told me.' Ok. Silence.

'So how are you?' At least she wants to know. Maybe.

'I've started painting again. I hear you book is going well.' More silence. 'Can we meet some time?'

'I'm very busy just now... but well, alright. Tomorrow at nine o'clock in the Old Toll. That's handy for you.'

'Fine, see you then.' We hung up. Mission accomplished. Lee and I went to the pub to celebrate. She bought me a drink. She took photographs of me looking scared. Looking sad. Looking over my shoulder just in case I had the night wrong. No, I am calm. We only went out for three years. I loved her and I am reasonably certain that she felt the same about me. We argued and never did get round to living together but we were close and I let her down. I let everyone down. Myself included. Not that I wanted to make amends exactly. Just explain. To tell the truth (which one should always endeavour to do unless it would be unwise). I had always been just a little afraid of Beck. Intimidated. She was so sorted. Everyone else we knew was such a shambling mess that she really stood out.

With the inexorable beat of time the next evening arrived. I had a cigarette with Lee before heading down the stairs to the pub, which was only two doors away. I was early. 'Better than being late,' I thought melodramatically, knowing that in one sense I nearly had been. Beck pushed through the door at exactly nine o'clock. The smile faded from my face as I saw the lack of one on hers. I left her to sit while I went to the bar. When I returned she looked into my eyes and said 'Well?' Unemotional, distant as the stars. I tried another smile.

    'How are you? How's work?' She looked away.

    'Yeah, not too bad. I've been made a partner in the practice.'

    'That's good. Security and all.'

    'I had thought I had that with you too.'

Flinching, I concentrated on separating the paper layers of the beer mat before replying.

    'I know. I'm sorry. I wanted to explain but now I'm not sure I can.'

'Are you that afraid of me? What can possibly change things for the worse here? I am only here because Lee badgered me. Said you'd changed – you seem pretty much the same to me.'

Fuck it. 'Ok. It's not pretty but I don't want sympathy. I just want you to know what happened.' I began my story.

It was a Tuesday. I remember that quite clearly. It was a Tuesday in January and it was dark and raining. The phone rang. Someone I did not know asked for me by name, and then asked about my relationship with James. I said he was my brother but we hadn't spoken for a while, maybe a few weeks. The stranger told me to get myself to Glasgow. Immediately, if possible. I felt my stomach plummet. I knew something was very wrong but the stranger would tell me nothing more over the phone. He told me to head directly to the Infirmary and ask for Dr Devlin as soon as possible. I called a taxi to take me to the station in twenty minutes – just in time to catch the last train. I threw my few meagre essentials into a rucksack. I thought of Beck and, as I scrabbled for a pen and some paper to leave her a note, the taxi's horn beeped outside. Scared and slightly panicky I ran for it, just made the last train. In Glasgow, I grabbed another taxi at the station there and sped off round the corner to the hospital. By that time, I was in too much of a state to notice that I probably could have walked there just as quickly. I ran to the information desk and asked for Dr Devlin. The clerk was startlingly efficient and had obviously been instructed to direct me immediately to Intensive Care. Intensive Care. Just the name made my head throb and my skin go clammy. Anyway, at a run I crashed through the ward doors to be confronted by a corridor with many other doors. A nurse stood outside one of these doors in conference with a tall man in a rumpled and ill-matched shirt and tie. He looked up, came towards me with a hand outstretched, introduced himself as Dr David Devlin. He said 'James is in here,' and showed me to a door. I hesitated. There could be no good outcome to opening this door. However, Dr Devlin ushered me into a small room overwhelmed with beeping, blinking machinery all attached to my brother by tubes. He looked pale and almost withered, as though the equipment was sucking the moisture from his body. Dr Devlin told me to be careful of the tubes and that James was drifting in and out of consciousness, that I should sit with him, could talk if I wanted but he could not reply because of the tube in his throat. I looked up at the doctor's tired face and mumbled a 'what?' 'He took an overdose of his medication. A man walking his dog found him on a beach at Loch Lomond. There can be effects on the heart, that's what these wires and this machine are. The problem is that we don't know how much he took or how long before being discovered he took it or if he took anything else. There's also the fact that he was found outdoors in the cold so it's basically a case of monitoring him carefully and waiting.' He checked a few machine screens. 'Is there anything you want to ask?' At that point, I could not even muster up any tears; I guess I was a little in shock.

> 'Why?' I searched the doctor's face for some kind of explanation.

He smiled gently.

> 'You'll have to ask him that. Is there anyone else we can call, he's only asked for you?'

I could only shake my head.

'Can I organise a cup of tea for you?'

What I felt like was a large whisky but, even in my shocked state, I realised I was not about to be offered that in a hospital. Dr Devlin left and, five minutes later, a nurse appeared silently and sat me down in the only chair in the stuffy room. She handed me a cup with a biscuit in the saucer and busied herself efficiently with the monitors. I sat there numbly all night and never did touch the tea.

Around six a.m. James stirred, looked into my eyes, tried to smile then closed his eyes again. A few minutes later first one, then another machine began squealing. I leapt up and pressed the call button but the door was already opening. Two nurses and a short woman in a white coat came charging into the room. They fiddled with tubes, wires, and the buttons on the monitors. The noise stopped.

'He saw me. He opened his eyes and saw me. What's happening?' One of the nurses ushered me gently out of the room.

Over the next few minutes, more staff came running in and out. I slumped on a chair in the corridor and waited.

The nurses left one by one. Then the doctor came out.

'I'm sorry,' she said quietly. 'We did everything we could.'

But he's only 32. He's too young to be dead. He just opened his eyes. How can anything so final have happened so quickly? I had no idea if I was just thinking these things or actually saying them aloud. The doctor took me to another room. I was brought another cup of tea. She explained that the strain on James's heart from the overdose of chlorpromazine had been too much and had finally caused a cardiac arrest. He had had a heart attack. Had I any idea why he would take such a large overdose? Was there anyone else they could call for me? They would have to do a post-mortem but I could spend a few minutes with him before they removed him to the mortuary. Did I know if he had made any plans in case of his death? They could put me in touch with an undertaker when the time came for such arrangements to be made. It all just washed over me at the time. There was no way I could take in the fact that James had looked at me then died. Almost as if that was what he'd been waiting for before letting go. Before letting go of life.

At that point, I suppose I should have called Beck. After all, she was a doctor and could help me deal with all of this, but it simply did not cross my mind. There was so much that did not make sense. So much left unexplained. So many questions without answers. I followed the doctor into James's room and pulled the chair over by the eerily silent bed. I held his hand and finally cried.

Later, of course, I hated him for putting me in this position. For waiting for me to arrive before dying. For almost laying the whole grim situation on me. Making me feel responsible somehow. That if I had not come running, he would have held on longer and might have recovered. But for the numb moments following his untimely demise all I could do was let the tears flow.

Led by Dr Devlin, I emerged from the room at around nine in the morning. Just when the rest of the world was starting its day, mine felt like I'd been on a weeklong bender. I was exhausted and emotional. I didn't know what to do. All I knew was that I couldn't go back to my quiet, settled life in Edinburgh without finding out more about James and what had driven him to his desperate last act. I did know that he had been under the care of a psychiatrist, that he was a schizophrenic. But everybody knew that. As a blood relative, the only remaining blood relative, how did I not know more? He would occasionally disappear off the radar for a few weeks at a time while he did his psychotic thing but he had always been back in touch once he was out of hospital or once the extra medication had kicked in. He had never liked me, or our parents when they had been around, visiting him in hospital. Always said he did not want us to see him when he was crazy. At some level, he must have known when he was, or perhaps it was just his paranoia stopping him letting us in. At his worst, when he let us visit in the early days, he would accuse us of all sorts of things. Stealing his thoughts, showing the aliens where he was. The aliens took the form of pigeons, so life must have been tough for him living in a city... Then our parents died in a car crash and even I had difficulty dealing with that, so how he coped I really did not know. I could not be there for him then – was barely there for myself. Beck helped me through that whole time. It must have been incredibly hard for him alone. Thinking about it now, even when everyone in the family was around, he had always been alone. We never really understood what his life was like, what went on in his mind. Now he was gone. Now it was me alone.

I booked into a backpackers' hostel by the river and went to a nearby old man's pub at opening time to toast James and the sadness and brilliance of his life. For about half an hour I was the only customer, but then the locals slowly began to arrive. Inauspicious entrances to their own private world of working all day to get drunk enough to face the night. I wondered if James had ever been like that – drinking away the day so that the night was bearable. Maybe he had even been to this bar. I sat with my double whisky and smoked cigarette after cigarette. Funny how the two go together. By late afternoon, I returned to the hostel and tried to sleep. Images of James's last look insistently came into my head. Had he wanted to say something? Was all he had wanted to see me one last time? I would never know. But what had happened in the last weeks of his life that had led him to such desperation? That I could try to find out. I resolved to begin the next morning by going to his flat. There might be some clues there I thought as I passed out into sleep.

James's flat was on the Southside in an old red sandstone tenement. I had only been there two or three times but I knew where it was and had his keys from the paltry personal effects given to me in the hospital. It was in immaculate order. I thought about my chaotic space and wondered at the hidden order in James's messy mind. In the kitchen, the dishes were all clean and in cupboards. I made a cup of tea and contemplated where to start. A note, perhaps. The computer was on the desk. There were no papers littered around it as there were around mine. There were, in fact, very few items to suggest personality. Few personal items. Not even many pictures on the wall. One of Loch Lomond though. The place must have meant something special to him if he chose that spot to die. I switched on his computer. There was a prompt for a password. First hurdle. I tried a few things that seemed relevant to no avail. 'Lomond' eventually unlocked the machine. The Loch again. The files were all as neat and ordered as his flat. There were folders for correspondence, work, writing and music. He had worked on a part-time basis as a graphic designer for a minor independent record label. He had written poetry and songs, played bass in a band who had recorded on the label he had worked for.

They had had minor success in the indie charts a few years back. Played gigs now and then around the student circuit. I wondered why he hadn't called anyone in his band, wondered again why he'd chosen me. A sudden sense of loss overcame me and I left the computer on and lay down on James's bed as grief washed through me. The tears at the hospital had been largely for me and from shock but finally I cried for him.

When I awoke, it took me a few minutes to work out where I was. James's curiously personality-free bedroom felt strangely homely. There, I felt more in touch with him and his life. Returning to his computer, I looked up his correspondence folder. I thought of my own files, all over the place. If I needed to reference something I had previously written, I had to take a guess at a file name and do a search for it. Once again, the orderliness of James's life astounded me. His letters were all in folders with the names of his correspondents and in date order. There were notes to a lawyer outlining changes to his will. All of his musical equipment and unfinished songs were to go to his band and everything else was destined for me. I looked around. There was not much. The fact that he had had so little to encumber him, so few possessions, made me cry again.

Examining the correspondence on James's computer led me to letters written to various people with our surname. Following links in the files showed that he had been looking into our family tree. There were census files going back to the early 1800s and letters to the registry office, which dealt with an area around the south of Loch Lomond where, apparently, our ancestors had settled in a village called Luss. I began to follow the same trails James had – looking back through the censuses at all the McFarlanes. There were generations of us going centuries back. There was a long line of McFarlanes. I found letters to some of these old relatives although they had been dead for 200 years. A particular John McFarlane seemed to have been the subject of most of the correspondence. He had lived in the 1700s – 1774-1807, his cause of death listed as 'melancholy'. From the letters, James seemed to have felt a particular bond to this man. He wrote to him as though he was a friend seen only last week. Conversational, eloquent letters to a good friend. There were even some responses, which I was alarmed to find until, reading them, I recognised James's style of writing. He had been corresponding with himself over 200 years. I began to realise just how fucked up James had been. Although the letters seemed very reasoned and rational, they were clearly an indication of the state of James's head.

John McFarlane was born in 1774 to a mother who was a crofter from Mull and a carpenter father from Fife, who had settled in the village of Luss on the banks of Loch Lomond so that the father could help build the church. John had grown up to be dux of the tiny school and become a poet and musician in the days when it was possible to choose poetry as a career. Unusually for those times, he had travelled all around Scotland in his 20s playing his music and reciting his verse. He cropped up in the census of 1801 in Arran. However, he had returned to Luss where he died in 1807 from 'melancholy', according to his death certificate. There had been a couple of volumes of his poetry published in the late 1700s, long out of print. Trawling James's bookshelves revealed that he had somehow managed to track down one of these volumes: 'A Book of Highland Verse'. Flicking through it quickly showed that it was standard fayre for the time, but James had obviously devoured the volume and read more into it than I did at first glance.

Therefore, in an effort to retrace James's state of mind, I settled down to read more. For days, I studied John McFarlane's history. From James's research and through his poetry, I began to develop an understanding of the man who had clearly been James's obsession before his death.

Dear John,

Although we are separated by two centuries, I feel I know you better than the family I have now. I, too, am a poet. I, too, play music and, although the genres are both very different, I feel you would understand me too. Like you, I took my music around the country and was sometimes welcomed, sometimes shunned, as I am sure you were. Not everybody understands art – it is not a universal truth. Unfortunately. Would be good if it were. I think then my life and yours would have been easier. I am speaking about my life as if it was over but, in a way, it is. I believe I have achieved all I can, said all I want to. I have left some moderately successful recordings and a collection of verse. Admittedly, the poetry has never been published, as yours was. But I have left it to be found after I am no longer around. Someone will find it. Maybe try for publication posthumously. At least, that is my hope and I have little hope left. In my opinion there is little left to hope for. The world's a fucked up place and I don't want to be a part of it any more. Having read your verse, I think you understood that too. I know you died of 'melancholy'. I know melancholy myself – melancholy is where I live. Not Glasgow. Not Scotland. It's where I would live wherever I called home. I have come to realise this over the years, as I'm sure you did. At brief intervals, I naively wished for more for myself, for my life, for my family and friends, but it was not to be. I can go no further. I am exhausted from all the years of trying so bloody hard.

Trying constantly and achieving nothing of note. But I have left something of myself. For some reason I feel that's important. Maybe because it provides proof that I was here at all. Maybe because I'm a typical, vain, self-important, weak human being. The latter seems more likely given the state of me and most of humankind. At least I had the dubious benefit of medical help for my melancholy, which I am certain you would have lacked. But all they really do, these medical 'helpers', is give me anti-depressants, anti-psychotics, anti-human drugs which make you 'better' by making you like everyone else. I never wanted to be just like everyone else. Again because I'm a vain, self-important excuse for a person. In some ways, I enjoyed being classed as mentally ill. It made me stand apart from the thronging mass of mediocre normality. It almost gave me an edge. Perhaps a vaguely dangerous edge. People in general are scared of difference, ergo, they were afraid of me. And (once again self-importantly) I liked that. But there comes a stage when that is no longer enough to sustain you. If you begin to live as the idea that others have of you, you inevitably begin to lose identity. You begin to be less true to yourself. I don't know why this truth is important but it certainly seems to be. Anyway. Back to medical treatment. (Although 'treatment' implies more than simple medication.) What happened to you in your melancholy? Were you just left to get on with it? I assume so. I also assume that you took your own life because, like me, you could not bear the horror of existence any longer. I really can understand that. It's exactly how I feel. Were you shunned in your village? The places you went to read and play. Did anyone take care of you? I can't find any mention of a wife in the research I've done. What did the doctors do to you in your time? For me, they find it helpful to lock me in with other crazy people every so often. I, for my part, don't find this helpful. I find this makes me worse. I find it allows me to pretend the remaining vestiges of 'normality', of sanity, can be transcended. When everyone around you is acting crazy, it marks you out if you're not. It's the opposite of society and societal living. When all those around you are yelling and screaming that they are the son of god, the longer you are there the harder it becomes to pretend that you're not the devil just for the fun of it. For a diversion. Of course, sometimes I have been the devil. Or, at least, the devil has been in me. I hear voices in my head. I only know they are in my head because I have been told this so frequently, because I have read up and done my own research. When these voices tell me things, they seem very real. I see things too. I have visions of destruction and death, which frighten me so much. If I'm walking over a bridge I visualise myself hurtling over the parapet to rivers or roads or railways underneath. If I'm crossing a road I visualise myself under the wheels of lorries and buses. If I'm just sitting in my flat I see knives flying towards me. Ok so the anti-psychotics help with this, but it all still happens. Right now, though, I am stable. I am thinking more clearly than I have for months. Maybe even for years. So why is it that now is the time I plan to kill myself? Because I know, it can't last. I know that, at some point in the future it will all happen again. And again. And I can't face going through all that even one more time.

So from me, John, it is hello and goodbye. If I believed in an afterlife, I'd believe we would meet there. Soulmates. Thank you for your poetry – I wish I could have heard your music.

Your distant cousin,

James

I guessed this was as close to a suicide note as I would find: James's last, and only complete, letter to John McFarlane. As it spewed from the printer I began to wonder why this man? What had been the connection James had imagined with this 200 year old relative? It did occur to me that the dates were similar, if separated by two centuries. A little further research looking into James's work on our family tree showed that John McFarlane had the same birthday as James, making James exactly two hundred years his junior. When I looked more closely at John's date of death, it turned out to be January 24th 1807 – exactly 200 years before I was called to see James at the hospital. The 1774 to 1807 replaced exactly by 1974 to 2007. They were the same age to the day when they died. I lay down on James's bed to contemplate this. Was this the connection? Had James planned his death to complete the pattern, the link?

I made the trip to Luss. It is a little village at the southern end of Loch Lomond. There are around fifty houses, a couple of tartan shops for tourists (of which there are many), two hotels, a pier and a church. In the churchyard, I found headstones for many generations of McFarlanes. John's was there. It read 'In loving memory of our son John' - again no mention of a wife, 32, single and melancholy. James all over. I sat on the shore, on the small pebbly beach and read John's book again searching for my brother. James had always been a troubled child, lonely even then. He did well at school, as did I, and while at fifteen I had been diagnosed as depressed, he had lasted until his early 20s before his behaviour became so bizarre that he was admitted to hospital in Edinburgh and we received the news that he was suffering from schizophrenia. Our parents were still alive back then and struggled to deal with first James, then I, being in the mental hospital.

Constantly wondering where they had gone wrong although, of course, it was not their fault. There was no blame to apportion, just a matter of faulty biology. They used to come into the ward to visit and bring us pizza. The hospital food was dreadful. Once I had been offered, as the vegetarian option, a baked potato with mashed potato filling. James tired first of their awkward and uncomfortable visits and asked the staff to stop them seeing him. I think, even in the depths of his psychosis, he felt self-conscious and instinctively strove for isolation rather than socialisation. On the other hand, I did not object to them coming in so they still had the opportunity to ask the staff about James whilst seeing me. Eventually when he was released back into the community, safe in shared sheltered housing with a CPN paying regular visits he became more willing to see us all. Although it is difficult to isolate yourself completely in a sealed hospital ward with nowhere to go other than the smoking room. Therefore, at first, I bore witness to his madness. All through this time, he had been writing and, in his spells out of hospital, had continued to play in his band. They were offered a contract to release an album on a small independent record label in Glasgow and shortly after that, James was offered a job there to design their covers. He moved through to Glasgow and we saw even less of him after that. He was very particular about his privacy and objected to other people's presence in his living space. When we met him, it was always on neutral ground in cafes and pubs. I felt slightly guilty that I had now pretty much moved into his flat – he would have hated that but, at the same time, he had put me in this position by calling me to witness his death. I felt I had little choice. Besides, I had made it my mission to understand his life and the end of it, so I needed to be where he had felt most settled, and I believed that meant necessarily straying into his space.

Footprints On The Moon

I walked along the shore in Luss, John's book in my bag. I stopped for lunch in a small café then returned to Glasgow. On occasion, Beck strayed into my mind but not to such a sufficient degree to inspire me to get in contact. I was a little adrift and had convinced myself that she would barely even notice my absence. When you are immersed in someone else's life, it is difficult to pay much attention to your own. In fact, I missed her less the more involved with James and John I became. It was only after my return some months later, that the magnitude of my neglect became apparent.

John walked into the small smoky room, a sheaf of papers under his arm. There was a gathering there, no spare seats. He stood at the fireplace and cleared his throat. Today was the day, the day he would make his name. He read smoothly and animatedly from his collection of poems. This was when he felt most comfortable in his own skin. This was what he knew best in his unsettled life. He read and people listened. There was even applause. He felt good. Tomorrow he would take his work to Edinburgh to be printed, but for now, he was happy with his progress. When he left the room to cheers and further applause, he decided to take a walk along the shore to the church his father had helped to build. He was 25 years old and on the verge of success. Of course, it was all relative. Already known around the Lowlands for his poetry and songs he had to venture further afield. John had never been further than Glasgow before and it was a daylong trip to get there. He borrowed a horse from one of his father's friends and left in the morning. On his arrival in Edinburgh four days later, he found his way to the public house where the literati of the day gathered. Insinuating his way into their company, he found a room in a boarding house not far from the Royal Mile. The Norloch was dirty and crowded unlike the loch he had left behind. He knew that within days, he would be homesick but he had a task to achieve before he could make the long journey back to Luss. The publisher accepted the money he had raised through his sponsors and set up the printing presses. John was to be a published poet. He sent his days courting the wealthy women who supported writers and they took him under their wings. They arranged for the distribution of his book and paid for further copies to be printed. Through these women, some copies even found their way as far as London. In his new guise as a successful poet, he began to tour around Scotland reading and singing. Well accepted wherever he read, he almost began to believe that his life was finally worthwhile but the melancholy was never too far away. It crept up on him in the most inauspicious circumstances and rendered him mute and bedridden. The doctors he could now afford seemed at a loss as to how to treat him and he was given potions and powders galore although none of them had much of an effect. In despair, he eventually returned to Luss where his parents took him in. Three days later, one January morning, he hanged himself from the lych-gate of the church his father had helped to build.

I walked into the small smoky room. There was a bar on the left and a haphazard array of battered copper-topped tables down the right. I bought myself a whisky and sat down in the furthest corner from the door. Lighting a cigarette, I took John's book out of my bag and started to read. At some point, a small piece of paper fell from between two pages covered with James's handwriting. This particular poem must have been special to him, must have meant something more than the rest of what was standard fayre for 18th century Scottish literature. The appearance of the note made me study that poem more in depth. It seemed to tell of a lonely life, a life lived in solitude and penury and this had sparked an interest in

James. His note read 'I know how you felt back then. I feel like that now. I have no-one and nothing.' This particular sentence hurt me – I had always tried to be there for him when he would let me, but I carried on reading. 'Despite my (very moderate) success as a songwriter and musician (and hopefully, posthumously, as a poet), I still feel all at sea as you say in this verse. I don't know what to do to change this, and I don't know if I want to. It is the way I have become accustomed to being over the years and I'm not sure I could cope with my life (and ultimately my death) in any other way. We have so much in common, you and I, that I can't help wondering why we could never meet. Perhaps we will later, although I don't really believe in an afterlife. What would you have made of my music and my words? They probably wouldn't mean that much to you. But I can read between the lines of your verses perfectly and I just want you to know that someone finally understands...' The note tailed off at this point. I believed it was the last thing James wrote. It was signed and dated two days before his death. Suddenly Beck and K sprang into my mind. 'I should call', I thought. Then I read the note again and the poem, and all thoughts of home left me. I left the pub in tears and retreated to James's monastic flat once more with little idea how I would carry on myself.

Apart from my rather flawed relationship with Beck, James had been my only remaining family. What was I going to do without him around any longer? We had hardly been close but we talked whenever we could and I was beginning to miss him terribly. When someone has shared memories, particularly those of childhood, their loss burns deeper than that of a more recently acquired acquaintance. Throughout our lives, James and I had been through so much together that with every passing minute after he had gone,

I was becoming more acutely aware of the depth of the loss I felt. In addition to his death, I was becoming lost in the mire of memory and grief and was finding it increasingly challenging to keep my own feet on the floor. It had been only four weeks since I had been called to James's bedside in the hospital. This time had taken its toll on my own health. I found myself barely able to drag my aching body from James's bed every day and then all I could face was whisky at the local pub. A diet of whisky and cigarettes does not make for optimal mental wellbeing as I well knew from my past, but seemed unable to alter. My old life in Edinburgh seemed further and further removed from my reality in Glasgow. Beck and all our unfulfilled plans seemed like nothing more than a distant dream, barely a memory, or so it felt. I knew I was slipping back into a depression but I didn't feel there was anything I could reasonably do to stop it. I was 34 years old and extremely tuned in to the signs. I registered with a medical practice near James's flat and made myself an appointment to see the doctor.

My gravity has loosened, relaxed its grip. I do not feel as bound to the earth as other people surely do, although, at the same time, I am feeling more and more pushed down. So much so that it is becoming difficult to move, even to breathe. I spend more and more time lying on James's bed staring at the artexed ceiling and drifting in and out of sleep. I have barely moved for some time...

Beck was still looking unimpressed by my story and even less impressed with me. I took a deep breath and continued...

Through my research on our family tree, following James's train of thought, I discovered that John MacFarlane had had a sister two years older as I was to James. I was almost afraid to look too deeply into her life in case there were similar parallels with us as there had been with James and John. With some sense of trepidation, I searched for Iona's death certificate. She had succumbed to a broken heart six months after John had passed away. Whilst my heart was broken now by James's last moments and the continued absence from my life of Beck or any contact with her, I was reasonably certain that in a few months I would have returned to what passed for normality in Edinburgh. I relaxed a little, believing that Iona's fate would not foretell my own, as John's seemed to for James. Iona, unlike me, had been a housekeeper for the local landowners. I could find no mention in the scant information I came across that she had had any leanings towards art. Housekeeping to me meant hoovering once a month and keeping the dishes clean - not at all my calling, not something at which I could have made my living. Although, to be fair, I did not really make anything like a living at art either. Yes, I had sold a few pieces, had some exhibited, but most had been given away to friends in return for favours. It was never commented on that the art's value would never compensate for the value of the favour done, always just polite acceptance that I had nothing more to give. At one stage during my time at art college when, it has to be said, I was more than a little crazy, I had thought to define myself in a painting. I worked day and night for months on this one canvas. I reasoned that, when it was completed, I would have no option but to kill myself having transferred all that I was into this work, until I realised that with every passing day, passing moment, I would have to add to it and I eventually abandoned it as unfinished. Sitting in James's flat now I wondered where that particular painting had ended up. More than likely stashed with the many other unfinished works in my studio to be painted over when I had run out of money for canvas. It had been a mess anyway.

Iona flexed her swollen knees as she bent down to sweep the remains of lunch into a dustpan. She wondered, not for the first time, how this had become her life - clearing up after the snobbish and uncaring Urquhart family. Just because they owned Luss and most of the surrounding farmland, that, in her opinion, did not make them better people than anyone else she knew. Admittedly, she did not know very many people, having lived her whole life in a tiny hamlet on the shores of Loch Lomond, but the ones whose acquaintance she had made seemed far more genuine and real than the almost mythical Urquharts. Only mythical in the sense that they were the equivalent of local royalty. Iona knew what went on behind the scenes and what they were really like and she was far from impressed by their wealth and notoriety. Her brother John had achieved his own small notoriety, which impressed her far more - he had made something of his life, been to Glasgow and Edinburgh, published poetry and songs. The fact that she had illustrated his book made her more proud than any of the mess in her day-to-day life at the Big House. She knew that her inauspicious etchings of lochside life had made it as far as London and her heart swelled with pride at what she and her brother had created. Iona loved John unreservedly, wishing eternally that he might be happier with his lot although, at the same time, she had to admit that she was not happy with hers. He got to travel doing what he loved and what he was good at whilst her days were passed sweeping up after an arrogant family she did not care about. If only it were possible for a woman to do what she loved and was good at for a living too. She would spend her time making her drawings and sitting on the pier sketching. Perhaps some work would come her way when John's book was read although she was sure her illustrations were largely unaccredited at the insistence of John's publishers. It was not an art book after all but one of verse. She sighed and eased her aching knees back to an upright position, wondering what John was up to at that moment and wishing she were anywhere else...

Leaving the new-found comfort of James's flat for the first time in days to attend my doctor's appointment, I explained what had happened, my history and how I felt. He prescribed me some anti-depressants and told me to return in a fortnight. I was not entirely surprised and went back to James's flat via the off-licence for some whisky and cigarettes knowing I would not feel any different in a matter of two weeks. Just had to bide my time waiting for the medication to kick in. On my return visit to the surgery, Dr Kerr referred me to a psychiatrist with a Community Psychiatric Nurse's support in the meantime. Karen-the-CPN was very helpful and a little concerned that I seemed to have immersed myself in my dead brother's life. Sequestered in his home and continuing his family tree research. Reading his books and, in essence, continuing where he left off. I had discovered that John MacFarlane's sister Iona, in a spooky but not entirely unexpected, coincidence, shared my birthday. There was almost a sense of inevitability about that. Nevertheless, I was determined that I would not complete James's imaginary connection. I expected that after a few months of anti-depressants I would be ready to return to face whatever remained of my old life in a different city. At one point I even lifted the phone to make contact with Beck but there was no answer. I realised that she probably would not recognise James's number and not call back, and that, it being a Saturday night, she would be out with all our friends. I felt a pang of regret that I was not there too but that was it – a momentary sensation, and I returned to sitting with my whisky reading John MacFarlane's poetry. I knew a lot of it by heart by then and it was beginning to mean more to me. It spoke of loss and longing and everyday life in a small village, which, by extension, was relevant to life in every corner of the world, simply concentrated in a smaller geographical area. I began trawling second hand and antiquarian bookshops in search of John's other volume with little success, not even knowing its title made seeking that particular book next to impossible. After two months and nothing, I found a friendly and helpful book dealer who looked up some obscure database and told me that the volume was entitled 'Lochside Life' and assured me he could track down a copy at a price. By that stage, I had very little money but I would have spent every penny if I could achieve my aim and further my immersion in James's obsession.

True to his word, within a month Robert had tracked down 'Lochside Life' and, true to my word, I gave him the last of my savings and retired eagerly to James's flat to read. I spent several days doing nothing but devouring poetry. By then I was familiar with John's style and immediately appreciated his work. With every stanza I felt I understood James more, losing more of myself in pursuit of James's reasoning, however flawed that may have been. It seems strange to me now that, as an artist, I barely noticed the illustrations in John's books, so intent was I on the words. When, finally they did strike me, it did not immediately occur to me that the I MacFarlane credited would be his sister Iona. Somehow, and rather embarrassingly, I simply assumed that a man must have done them. Through further reading around the history of the time they lived, it seemed unlikely that a lowly housekeeper, and a woman at that, could produce such masterful sketches let alone have them reproduced in published works. Even the terminology: 'masterful', suggests masculinity. Therefore, it was quite a shock when I read the fine print at the back of 'Lochside Life' and discovered that Iona had been the artist. There was a connection between her and I after all. Two hundred years after her artistic endeavours had gone largely unnoticed, mine had too. I logged on to James's computer and began composing a letter to Iona, fully aware that I was following James's example too closely. But still certain that I would end up fine despite the fact that I was crying every day for all my accumulated losses and, however much whisky I consumed and however many anti-depressants I swallowed, I was not feeling any better. Karen the CPN was becoming increasingly concerned about my isolation and seeming obsession and had fast-tracked the appointment with the psychiatrist which was now only three weeks away.

Dear Iona,

You were born 200 years to the day before me yet I feel we are connected by more than distant blood. You were an almost secret artist and I, for my part, am largely unfulfilled in this sphere. Whilst I went to college and studied for four years, I doubt you could even read or write but you could draw. You expressed yourself. I too have spent my life attempting to express what I feel via the medium of paint. At least your work was reproduced and could be widely seen during your lifetime, a goal that has so far eluded me. I know your younger brother ostensibly achieved more whilst he was alive as did mine. I know you loved him and did not begrudge his successes. I feel the same about mine. Felt. Past tense now. Our brothers died at exactly the same age and you only have a few months left to live. No offence, but I am determined that I will break the connection. The parallels between all our lives will end with me. I almost wrote 'will die with me' but then realised that would fulfil an unspoken prophecy. Yes, right now, my heart is broken, but I remain optimistic that this will heal with time and I will not die imminently. I have still not completed my defining artwork. The fact that I have not touched a paintbrush let alone stretched a canvas for over six months notwithstanding. Also I believe that until I have created my definition I still have more to say. Like footprints on the moon, my achievement will remain forever in a world that has long forgotten me. I become more resolute in this belief with every passing day. The drugs I am on will help me. The psychiatrist will help me. Karen-the-CPN will help me. Perhaps even my erstwhile friends will help me when I eventually return to my old life. Which I intend to do once my heart has mended.

Did you witness your brother's death? I did mine. That is why I am such a mess at the moment. However, this state of affairs will change. It will just take time and, as I do not think for a moment that I will die too on the day that you did, time is something I have. I will be in touch after I've seen the consultant.

Signing off for now.

Dear Iona

I have seen the psychiatrist now. There were no such professionals in your day. Otherwise, John might have survived his melancholy. Although, to be fair, they didn't stop James losing his battle with the same affliction. James left me in charge of his poetry. I have sent some to a few modern day publishers and am waiting to hear from them. 'Poet' is not really an achievable thing to be these days. Not if you want more reward than integrity. James was known a little in his time as a songwriter and musician. Like your brother, he toured to showcase his creations. Even made a little money at it although I believe it was the craft of writing he loved more than the performing. He had always been a shy child. Very bright, very intelligent, but shy. I think when he played in his band he could put on a persona and pretend he was someone else. Was your brother like this too? Or did he enjoy giving readings? I only saw James on stage a handful of times. He did not like people he knew well to watch, I think because he became his alter ego rock star. He wasn't too keen on us even seeing him in his normal crazy state. I think he was lonely. I was too, even though I was in a seemingly stable relationship. Did you have a significant other? I can find no mention of this in the little information I have discovered about you.

Anyway, as I said, I have seen the psychiatrist now. I did not tell her about you, or John. I only mentioned my own brother and the fact that now he has gone I have no-one. She suggested a short stay in the hospital but I know what that means – I've been there before. It means being locked away with a bunch of other nutters and becoming more unhinged by the day. I said no thank you. She said to bear it in mind as though my mind will change. I'm not at that stage right now. Never say never but well, never again as long as I have a choice in the matter. Right now, I will make do with the occasional consultation and regular meetings with Karen-the-CPN. I want to ask how you die of a broken heart but I am afraid of the answer…

Signing off for now.

I sit opposite Beck in the pub and realise it's nearly closing time. She retains a reasonably hard and unmoved expression whilst I have been animated and tearful throughout my story. I wonder whether she ever really loved me. If so, how could my tale not be having an effect? 'Last orders,' the bartender shouted, ringing the bell.

'What do you want to do?' I asked Beck.

'I have to go home. Working in the morning,' she replied with an unreadable expression.

'But I still have more to tell you,' I almost whined.

Her face twitched into something like a grimace, but she took a deep breath and then said 'Ok, I'll come up to Lee's for a little while.'

I expected a 'for old time's sake' or something else asinine that never came for which I was immensely grateful. We finished our beers and retired to Lee's sitting room, opening up another couple of bottles. It bothered me that she seemed so unemotional but I reminded myself that she was a doctor and probably heard crazy shit all the time. Perhaps I was foolish to expect that, just because we had been together a while back, she still cared. I did. Too embarrassed to admit that, I simply continued with my tale…

Iona MacFarlane took to her bed three months after her brother John's death. She could no longer face sweeping up or changing the beds of the Urquharts. Realising that she would become a penniless drain on her own family made her feel bad but at least they cared and would continue to look after her as she wallowed (as she felt she was doing) in her sorrow. She had stopped drawing on the day she was taken aside by the lady of the house and told the news of John's death. Her immediate instinct had been to run to his side and shake some sense into him. He was doing well for a poor boy from a small village – he had made a name for himself all over the country. She wished she had been the one with the affliction of melancholy instead of him. Perhaps she would have been able to appreciate the love of those around her and, more importantly, to keep going, to remain alive. Even the sparkle of spring sunshine on the loch she loved could not inspire her to move let alone draw. Sighing, she turned over in her small bed and attempted one more time to get the rest she knew would not come.

It was summer and, oddly for Scotland, the sun had come out. I awoke with a sense of dread I could not explain until I realised it was the 28th of July – my birthday (and Iona MacFarlane's). It was difficult to breathe. I called Karen-the-CPN although when she answered I had nothing to say. She said she would come round in the afternoon. That seemed such an unfeasibly long time to wait. I knew I would not be able to get back to sleep so I showered and made some coffee. In a fit of restlessness, and not knowing how else to pass the time, I cleaned James's flat from top to bottom, returned all the dishes to their respective cupboards, dusted the bookshelves and the computer, changed the bed sheets and hung out a wash in the tenement garden. Exhausted, I sat down at the desk and printed out my letters to Iona, as well as those James had written to John. I felt that it was time to come clean with Karen-the-CPN. So far, I had kept our distant relations and present-day relationships with them from her. It was such a big part of my life that it had been extremely difficult to remain silent all this time but I felt that today was the day I would finally be honest with her about the depth of our obsessions. I composed one last letter to Iona…

Dear Iona

It is our 35th birthday, separated by two hundred years but still. Happy birthday. I'm not having such a good one myself. I feel crushed by the effort of breathing, of having to remain upright. I received no cards this morning. I have nobody left who either knows or cares that I have reached a milestone. Or should that be millstone? It certainly feels like there is a massive and immovable weight around my neck. There is only one way out as far as I can see with my limited vision. Today I break the curse, or whatever it is, we have between us. This is the end...

Signing off for good.

With uncontrollable tears streaming down my face, I printed out my last letter and poured a large whisky. Over the last fortnight, I had been stockpiling painkillers – buying no more than one packet a day in order to allay suspicions in the pharmacy. I sat down in James's armchair and took them all, washed down with whisky.

The buzzer rang an hour later. I had forgotten about Karen-the-CPN's imminent visit. Or perhaps I hadn't and was really waiting for her to arrive. Almost reluctantly, I let her in. She took one look at me, the Paracetamol paraphernalia surrounding my chair and hustled me down the stairs to her car. In my compromised state, I was unaware of where we went, which roads we took, but I am sure that Karen-the-CPN was breaking all sorts of speed limits. We screamed into the hospital car park and I was rushed inside and put on a trolley. She followed me in and explained to a very nice doctor what I had done and I was wheeled away into a room where a variety of staff busied themselves around me. Karen-the-CPN held my hand as they pumped warm water down a tube in my throat into my stomach.

I had never felt so bad before. I could not stop crying. Karen-the-CPN stayed with me until I had stopped throwing up and waited with me until they came to wheel me into a ward where a grumpy balding man spoke to me for a while. Then I was put to bed with a charcoal drink and Karen-the-CPN left. I was not sure but I was fairly certain I was locked in. Eventually I succumbed to sleep.

When I awoke, confused and still crying, a nurse brought me a cup of tea. My head felt fuzzy and my throat hurt. I asked her where I was and what had happened. Her reply did not shock me. I was indeed in a locked psychiatric ward and a doctor would be in to see me soon. For the first time in six months, I felt as though I could abdicate from the responsibility of being. I was not alone. It was almost a relief. Probably would have been had I not felt so wretchedly miserable. As promised, a doctor appeared at my bedside and spoke to me in a soothing voice. A nurse took some blood and smiled gently at me, patted my arm as she left. The doctor, who seemed younger than me, said that I would be moved in the morning to the local psychiatric hospital under section once the blood test results had come back. They were checking to see if I had damaged my liver, as is apparently common practice after a Paracetamol overdose. Somewhat inconsequentially, I wondered what would happen to the washing I had hung out on the line. I must remember to ask Karen-the-CPN about it, I thought to myself. I fell back into a restless sleep.

Inevitably and inexorably morning came. I was dimly aware that there was sunlight beyond the dusty windows. A cheery orderly brought me some toast and tea. A different doctor came with Karen-the-CPN and asked me how I felt which just seemed like such a woefully inadequate question. He said they had pumped my stomach in time for there to be minimal effect of the pills on my liver but that they were putting me on a Short Term Detention Order under the Mental Health Act Scotland. For a period of four weeks from today, I was to be confined in the nearby psychiatric hospital under supervision. Forms were signed and I am sure other things happened of which I remained unaware, but the outcome was that Karen-the-CPN drove me to another ward in a different place and left me there. Abandoned me there, it felt like. I was in a strange city where medical professionals were the only people I knew. And, whilst I had been in hospitals before – many times in fact, that had all been in Edinburgh where I had a support network and even got to know some of the other regular patients. Here in Glasgow I was totally alone. At that point, I missed Beck and the gang more than ever. Particularly Beck. But I was too much of a mess and too afraid to call. By that point, it had been over six months since I had been in contact and I could well imagine the fallout situation from a desperate and pleading message now. Therefore, I took to my bed and followed instructions and never did find out what happened to my washing.

Somehow, with a strict regimen of hiding in my cubicle and doing what I was told, I survived my four weeks. Various meetings were held where doctors, nurses, and Karen-the-CPN discussed me as though I was not present and eventually I was allowed out. I took a taxi back to James's flat, not knowing where the hospital was and, exhausted, slept for two days.

Karen-the-CPN came round and I told her I felt I needed to reconnect with my old life. Moreover, I needed to paint and had no means of doing that where I was. Reluctantly, she agreed that I should take a couple of days to return but that she wanted to see me after that, which seemed reasonable to me. I packed my few meagre possessions into my rucksack and made my way to Queen Street Station. It felt as though I had been gone rather longer than a mere seven months – so much had happened in that time that the world and my place in it had forever altered.

I was nervous on the train, not certain what I would find at the other end of the line. Arriving at Waverley, I slowly walked up the hill to the bridge before, finally, the realisation struck me that I was not ready for this. I wandered aimlessly for a short while around a town still thronging with festival crowds, before boarding a bus to Gullane, needing more time to prepare myself.

It was a warm day and the air was still...

Eileen M Taylor

Footprints On The Moon

THE CARRIER

Eileen M Taylor

1

It was early on that Tuesday when I arrived in The Hod Carrier – not yet lunchtime. There was nobody else there. Just me and Damon, who was standing at the end of the bar smoking. 'What do you want?' he mumbled, reluctantly stubbing out his cigarette and easing his way behind the counter. I ordered my usual pint and rolled a cigarette of my own. He moved off to the end of the bar again to read the sports section whilst I was attempting to start my brain working. It was our morning ritual. Almost every day began this way. Once he'd finished reading about his team's latest defeat and I'd kick-started my head, we'd chat and bitch and smoke together for several hours. The bar was usually near enough empty during all this. Only around mid-afternoon did the majority of its other punters start arriving. Even then, in a street full of packed pubs, the Hod was pretty quiet. I could almost invariably park myself on 'my' stool at the end of the bar for as long as I wanted. To be fair, it was a particularly poor pub with a reputation as somewhere to get more drunk when other bars wouldn't even serve you. I only really went there because I liked the staff. Although the fact that it was quiet and slightly disreputable also appealed for the obvious reason that so was I. It only took a matter of weeks from moving into my flat around the corner to knowing the regulars at the Carrier – a few rookie mistakes quickly establishing the ones to talk to and the ones whose eyes must never be caught, and even the nuances of facial expression which meant avoiding the reasonably sane ones, at least for a couple of pints. Of course, in a pub like the Carrier, sanity, like the beer, is a fairly free-flowing concept. Still there is a strange, and, indeed, strangely comforting, sense that however shit a time you're having, someone else in the same room has had worse. Much worse. At least, I used to think that. Now I'm not so sure...

Damon and I were filling random letters into the crossword when the old boy came in. We never knew his name, not his real one at any rate, not at that stage, but we called him Dirk because of his relentless (yet unconscious) Scottishness. Every town in Scotland has a Dirk. He is the one who wears a jimmy-hat without any sense of irony, or, it would seem, self-awareness, a kilt even though he is so painfully skinny that it's a constant worry he's going to lose it. And it's most definitely not for the tourists. He will not leave his hostel without full national dress (sans skean dhu, mercifully) – whatever the weather, whatever the occasion. We do take the piss a little, Damon and I, but Dirk seems to neither notice nor care. In a way I guess I quite admired his total lack of concern as to what others thought or said of him. Although sometimes the stories he told (during his rare lucid moments) of his younger days even brought tears to Damon's eyes. To be fair though, he really was just a diversion for us. Damon, in his role as care-in-the-community barman, couldn't really afford to invest too much in any of his patrons, although he seemed to have made an exception for me. And, well, I'm just either too shallow to give a fuck, or too easily influenced. Whichever – neither are 'qualities' to take any pride in.

Anyway. Dirk sat on his own nursing his pint for a while. He seemed oddly pensive, a little resigned. Or perhaps that's just my attempt at spin – a revisionist history to make it all less bewildering, less frightening. In any case, he wasn't agitated, nor was he incoherent, he just sat quietly. We ignored him and laughed as we made up words which fitted in with all the wrong ones we'd already put into the grid and couldn't be bothered to change. I ordered another pint. We smoked some more.

When the door crashed open it must have been around quarter to two. Some young lad fell inwards, covered in blood. At first we couldn't tell where he was hurt, or even if it was his own blood. But, as Damon started towards him, we saw the knife. I ducked round behind the bar. I'd like to say that I was heading for the telephone, that I was leaping, in my non-confrontational way, to my friend's defence, but that would be a lie. I was just shit-scared, saving my own skin. Some of what happened over the following few minutes is a bit vague as I only heard and did not witness, and, of course, I'm sure I've rationalised much of it from the safe perspective of the present so that those few instants of the past make more sense.

Apparently it wasn't Damon the young guy was aiming his vicious gaze (and knife) at – it was Dirk. Whatever was going on, from what I was aware of, there had been nothing previously which would have suggested trouble. In all the shouting voices I definitely heard Damon trying his psychologist's talking down tactics. I'd heard that so many times before as the various psycho regulars had gone off on one. It seemed that the young guy's mates followed him in and they surrounded Dirk, who I never heard say a word. There was yelling – accusatory and malicious – then an eerie wet gurgle, then silence. The door crashed open again. A flurry of footsteps. Then nothing. Nothing for several moments until I heard a sob which, I discovered later, was Damon. He called my name and suddenly I realised I was still crouched on the floor, unseen, behind the bar. I grabbed the phone to the floor and dialled 999, still too scared to look. Once the police and an ambulance had been summoned, I stood up.

When I saw what... when I could take in what lay in front of me, I'm ashamed to say I threw up. Dirk lay in a spreading pool of blood which even the already tacky red carpet would not disguise. Damon stood over him, shirtless. Attempting to stem bleeding from various places with his work clothes. I swallowed, braced myself, grabbed as many bar towels as I could, ran to Damon's side. Blood bubbled from Dirk's mouth with a sad damp sound as I felt for a pulse. I couldn't find one. I couldn't even try CPR with all that blood. Damon and I sat down away from Dirk, in the blood, and couldn't meet each other's eyes. When it had come down to it, he'd stepped up and I'd hidden. The realisation of just how different we really were is something we've never talked about, but never quite forgiven me for. Neither of us.

The ambulance arrived first. Paramedics running in their green overalls. Not their job to be judgemental, just to preserve life. They moved Damon and I out of their way and set about Dirk with admirable efficiency. Without really knowing what else to do, Damon and I went back to sit at the bar. He poured himself the largest whisky I've ever seen. We said nothing. The crossword seemed such a stupid thing to have been so involved in now. When the police arrived and cordoned off the whole pub, the paramedics hoisted Dirk onto a stretcher and rolled him away. We were questioned, taken to the station and questioned some more. I was finally dropped home at 2a.m. My flat seemed empty and too quiet. I put on the loudest, most aggressive music I could find, risking, uncaring, the wrath of my neighbours. They've never liked me anyway. Always hoping I'll leave and not bring down the tone of the place any longer. They're all lawyers and doctors and MSPs and professors and I'm, well, nothing. I'd always been perversely proud of my nothingness, knowing that inside it wasn't the case. But that night... Never in my life had I felt so worthless. Useless. Pathetic. I think I was almost hoping one of the other residents would knock on my door to complain so that I could tell them what had happened. As if that would make it more real to me too. But no-one came. I just lay on my floor in the blast of music and cried.

2

I lay on the floor for a long time. Outside time was still passing, the world was still turning. I could tell from the movement of light through my window, noises in the street. After what must have been several days even I could not bear to hear the same cd on constant repeat any longer. I remember it as one of the hardest things I have ever had to do to leave the flat. I took the extremely long way round to reach my local shop for cigarettes to avoid passing the Carrier. Damon and I had not been in contact at all. I assumed that, like me, he was numbly confused and scared. But I had the added burden of shame.

For a few days after that I craved silence. The sort of silence it is impossible to find in a city centre block of flats. I contemplated getting on a train. To anywhere up north where I could see the stars. I contemplated throwing myself from my 4th floor window to achieve the ultimate silence. To finally escape the violent self-loathing. But I did neither. What I did was lie on the floor some more. It reminded me of a poem I'd written as a troubled teen: 'lying on the floor/ 'cos you can't get any lower/ without being in the ground'.

It was the longest I had been without a drink for many years.

In the end though, I had to move. This time I did, tentatively, approach the Carrier. The police tape had gone, of course it had. There were people inside. I pulled the door open.

Damon wasn't there, it was Kevin behind the bar. In a way I was relieved, although I felt that Damon and I needed to talk. Or rather, I needed to talk to him. I had no idea what to say, how to even venture a 'hello', but nobody else had been there, experienced what we had...

Although the carpet had been replaced there was always going to be an area of that pub in which I could never again stand. I just kept picturing the floorboards below stained forever with Dirk's blood. Blood stained everything I saw whether my eyes were closed or open. The customers obviously had heard some version of events and looked away as I sat down and ordered a pint. Kevin at least made an attempt to be polite. 'How you doin'?' he said. 'Ok' was all I could muster as a response. He was desperate to ask me questions but unsure as to how to broach the subject for which I was grateful. I couldn't even finish my pint. Left in a silent storm of unasked questions, a sense of envy I knew I didn't deserve, and a sense of blame I thought I did.

I knew I would not be back there.

3

Away from the Carrier I attempted to put my life together, to make things make sense to me. I realised that for this to happen I needed to know more about Dirk (who by then I'd found out was called Hamish Sutherland). Finally I took a chance and called Damon. We arranged to meet the following day in a pub far from the Hod.

I arrived early – I've always been obsessively early – bought myself a pint and sat down in the furthest, quietest corner of the dim, smoky bar. Almost inexplicably I was nervous. Damon was a long-standing friend. Surely he, out of all the long-standing friends I knew, would not be as judgemental as I was myself. Surely I had no need to feel anxious. Surely this meeting couldn't be as bad as the countless variations of it I had imagined in the preceding weeks...

When he walked in exactly on time I thought he looked exhausted. I suppose I did too – I certainly hadn't been getting my eight hours a night since... the incident. I smiled a tentative hello, testing the ground. He gave an insincere grin back but appeared pleased to see me. I went to the bar: acquired pub etiquette – first one there buys the first round and, being compulsively early, it's always me. We sat in silence for a while, neither sure how to begin. In the end it was Damon, once again, who stepped up.

'How've you been, you look tired?'

'You too,' I smiled. 'I guess I'm ok. I'm still here at least.'

He nodded as though he too felt almost guilty about that.

'I'm sorry.' I had the beginnings of tears in my voice and eyes.

'Yeh, me too.'

'I mean I'm sorry about...'

'I know. There was nothing you could've done anyway.'

'Still...' I wiped angrily at my face. 'I've felt so bad. About everything.'

We sat in silence again until we'd both stopped crying long enough to laugh at each other.

'What the hell are we gonna do?'

'I need to know. Why, how, what the fuck happened. That poor old guy...' I put my glass down and cleared my throat. 'You heard his stories too. Was there anything there? Anything that would shed some light on all of this? I mean, I assume the police asked you about him. They asked me too but he'd just been this crazy old guy we made fun of...' I was talking too much but the confusion which had been my life for the last month was in full spate. Damon calmed me with a look, my voice had been becoming louder. In an effort of will just sufficient to prevent me from being exiled from another pub, I quelled my rising hysteria and lowered my voice so much that Damon had to lean in to hear me. 'I just keep seeing that stupid jimmy-hat on the floor beside him... you know... after... I wonder where it went. Did he have any family any more? Or real friends? Has anyone missed him? I don't know why but I need to know and all I've got are his stories and his name.'

'I'm not sure how true his stories were, and I'm sure we both heard the same ones. What are you trying to prove?'

'I'm not trying to prove anything. I just need to make sense of this.'

'You'll just make yourself crazy. Leave it to the police.'

'But it's been over a month now and they've got nothing. I read the paper every day and there's no mention of Dirk. Nobody's been caught. Nobody really knows why a sad, lonely old guy was killed and nobody really cares. I was there. We were there. Don't you want to know?'

'I think I really want to forget about it and get on with my life but I know I won't. I know it's not something you can just let go of, but you have no idea what you're doing. And if the police can't find anything how on earth are you going to?'

I hung my head, exhausted. I knew he was right but I couldn't give up now that I'd built some kind of purpose into my life. What I really wanted was for him to help me but he was not my therapist. He was not the police. He was a barman who'd witnessed something terrible. He got up to leave.

'Stop before you get in too deep. Or before you find you can't find anything and feel crap. I know that's what you'll do. Yes, you've been through something awful but how is gnawing away at that going to help you move on?'

He said he'd see me soon but I couldn't tell whether that was just how he said goodbye or if he meant it.

4

At the time of his death Hamish Sutherland had been 70 years old – the same age as my grandparents. However, unlike my grandparents, comfortable in suburbia with their tea and their potplants, he'd spent the last years of his life wandering around the city and sitting in pubs, often the Carrier though he had frequently been sighted elsewhere, telling tales from his past or just keeping quiet and ignoring the jokes he neither seemed to know nor care were inevitable. All we knew for certain about him was that he lived in a hostel near the Grassmarket, he wore his full traditional wardrobe every day and he drank a half pint of heavy with a nip of whisky. He had never been a troublesome customer, tiresome occasionally, but usually by the time he was done with his storytelling he'd have had enough drink and leave of his own accord. Of course, lacking a certain sense of self-awareness meant that frequently he would start talking in the midst of another conversation or (a cardinal sin in a Scottish pub) while the football was on. But mostly he kept to himself and didn't bother anybody. I forced myself back to the day it happened, imagined myself crouched behind the bar, tried to recreate the scene in my mind. What had been yelled? Was there some clue there? Surely one of the lads had let something slip in the anger and adrenalin of the moment. Certainly there had been some swearing... But my memory was flawed and I could not recall anything with any great clarity. I had to concede that this was not a promising start to making sense of Dirk's death. Damon's words echoed round the empty cavern of my head: 'what if you can't find anything... you'll make yourself crazy.' I was making myself crazy just sitting in my flat every day knowing nothing anyway.

There had to be something else I could do.

It was a Friday five weeks after Dirk's death. I left my flat without a plan and went wandering.

5

The Grassmarket pubs were busy with lunchtime workers and tourists, but I found a seat in the beer garden of the Beehive. Of course I'd wandered here – subconsciously I had known that this was where I was heading but, now that I was here, I realised I had no idea of what I was seeking, how to proceed. Silently I sipped my warm lager and smoked to keep the wasps away as I considered my next move. There were hostels all over this part of town and I had no idea which one Dirk had stayed in, but there were bound to be others in similar situations to his nearby who may or may not talk to me. It wasn't much but it was a possible starting point. At least it gave me an initial aim as I carried my empty glass back to the bar and walked out into the thronging street.

The Grassmarket is a strange mix of pubs, hostels and hotels and has an equally eclectic mix of shops from those selling high-end musical equipment to ethnic bargain stores. I headed for the Cowgate end at the foot of Greyfriars Street and struck up a conversation with the Big Issue seller on the corner.

'How are you today?' I ventured optimistically.

'Aye, can't complain,' came the slightly suspicious reply.

'Do you stay around here?'

He pointed a nicotine stained finger at the hostel directly opposite where we stood.

'Been there long?'

'Long enough.'

'Did you ever know a Hamish Sutherland?' I asked hopefully.

'Might have.' He shifted his feet uncomfortably, gave me an odd look.

'Did he live there with you?'

'Look, what do you want?'

'I'm just trying to find out about him. I knew him a little...'

'Yeah, well, I didn't.' His face closed off. 'I haven't got anything else to say to you.'

I smiled brightly, said thank you and crossed the street, clutching my newly purchased Big Issue.

After two more frustratingly similar abortive conversations, I returned to the Beehive to regather my thoughts. It seemed evident that I was approaching this the wrong way. So far nobody had wanted to offer me any information – where was I making mistakes? I realised with a startle that the men I had spoken to probably thought I was some kind of do-gooder whereas, and this came in a further wave of shock, I was in fact doing something completely self-serving. Unsure as to which was worse, I gave up my quest and took the long route home.

The following day I awoke with a new sense of purpose. I visited a cash machine and returned to the Grassmarket, retracing my steps. Nodding to yesterday's Big Issue seller, I continued on up the hill to Greyfriars churchyard. There was usually a crowd from the hostels who hung about the side door of the Bedlam Theatre, drinking out of sight of their residences. I stood nearby and lit a cigarette, working out my best approach. A stilted 'do you mind if I join you?' seemed altogether too formal and Christian. I didn't want them to think I was about to start handing out tracts about how the lord would save them and help them repent their sinning ways. The thought almost made me laugh out loud. In the end I went to the off-licence round the corner and bought a crate of lager and simply sat down with them. I introduced myself and their initial suspicion was allayed when I handed round the beers. Gradually they resumed their conversations. I didn't say much but just enough for them to begin to include me. Big Jim seemed to be the group's leader. Everyone else stopped and listened when he spoke. By the end of the afternoon after many beers we were all quite merrily friendly. When I left I shook Big Jim's hand and didn't let on that I was returning to my own flat. I felt a little duplicitous but simultaneously, and quite surprisingly, admitted to myself that I had actually enjoyed my day.

For the next couple of weeks my days all followed the same pattern. I'd join Big Jim, Davey, Mikey, Bob and Helen on the bench for a few or more of the beers I'd take along. I never once mentioned Dirk in that time and I began to realise that I had more in common with these people on the fringes of society than I had with any of the very select few from school or university with whom I'd kept in touch. Each day I began to look forward to my session a little more. It made me feel underhanded and guilty on the rare occasions I remembered what my purpose in getting to know this group was. Eventually, I knew I would have to start my Dirk conversation. As it happened, I didn't need to...

6

Big Jim cleared his throat and began to speak.

'Steaming,' he said, his voice rumbling out of him like molten rock from an eruption. Everyone stopped and regarded him carefully.

'What?' I asked, unsure as to whether he was simply referring to his current status.

'That's what killed Hamish. A gang steaming.'

My blood ran just a little colder suddenly as I realised this was what I'd been waiting to hear all these weeks.

'What's that?' My voice came out as a separate entity, recalcitrant and cracking.

'Bunch of kids get high, take to the streets armed with whatever and stab their way around until they get caught or come down...' He paused, took a long swallow of his lager and looked around for confirmation from the others.

Davey and Bob nodded sagely.

'It's bad,' ventured Helen, 'a big problem.'

'I've never heard of it before,' I said in my choked voice.

'That's because you've led a sheltered life.' Big Jim had a wicked glint in his eyes as he continued. 'Living in your fancy West End flat with your posh front door and your education.'

I felt my heart drop into my abdomen and my face turn crimson.

I stuttered 'how...? What?'

'Aye, we've been onto you for a while. Figured you had some secret agenda, some sort of reason for hanging out here with us. Mikey followed you one night. Saw you go into a block on Chester Street.'

I stared at the ground, studied my beer can, looked anywhere but at Big Jim. He laughed, a hollow sound with no humour and a touch of maliciousness.

'So what is it? Were you the one who witnessed Hamish's death?'

Slowly, I nodded silently.

'It's been driving me crazy,' I croaked nervously. 'There was no news, no word from the police. I needed to find out something and I didn't know how.'

'So you found us?' Bob said quietly.

'I think you underestimated us,' Big Jim rumbled.

I nodded again, embarrassed beyond words.

"However,' he continued, 'we reckon you can get back to your comfortable life now that we've told you what you wanted to know.'

I could feel tears of shame pricking at my eyes. 'But...'

'You don't belong here with us,' Big Jim uttered with finality. He looked away as if dismissing me.

'You don't understand,' I managed to make my voice heard amidst their laughter. Big Jim fixed me with his piercing and surprisingly clear blue eyes.

'Well? If you can make me understand I might just see my way clear to keep speaking to you.'

'I'm just like you. I've never fitted in with my neighbours. I don't really have any friends to speak of. These last weeks have made me feel like I finally belong somewhere...' I faltered as I gazed round at their faces regarding me with almost scientific interest. 'And, yes, I do have a posh address but that's not where I feel at home – this is.'

'Well listen, kiddo, whatever you do isn't going to bring Hamish back.'

'I know that, I just thought...'

'Hear me out,' insisted Big Jim. 'In a way I admire what you're trying to do and I'd help if I thought I could. Don't ever like hearing one of our own has gone however it happens. But with Hamish, you're just going to have to accept that that's it. The police hardly ever find these gangs and even if they do it's all conjecture, they can't find any evidence.'

'But I have to know more...'

'Why? Just leave it kiddo. It won't do you any good.'

With echoes of Damon's words in my head, I stood up, finally angry.

'What is it that nobody wants me to find out?' I exploded, to Big Jim's obvious surprise. 'Hamish wasn't exactly a friend but I knew him and I watched him die. Why can't anyone understand that I need to find reasons...?'

I ran out of steam as Helen put her arm around me.

'Listen love,' she almost whispered, 'it's over. Just accept that and move on. Go home.'

Davey and Bob nodded silently. Big Jim softened his voice, 'Helen's right and you know that really. Take my word for it, kiddo, no amount of your amateur detective work will make the slightest difference. Go home and get on with your life.'

Finally accepting defeat, I turned and walked away.

7

Three months to the day after Dirk's death, I woke up woolly mouthed in my own bed wondering what to do next. Being warned off my investigations firstly by Damon, then by Big Jim, only served as to make me more determined to continue. But how? Where would I turn? In an exercise in vain optimism over hope I called the local police station, asking to speak to the officer who had questioned me after the incident. After an interminable wait listening to Greensleeves over and over and being bounced between departments, PC Shaw finally came on the line.

'Hello,' she said. 'What can I do for you?'

'It's about Hamish Sutherland's case,' I began somewhat tentatively. 'I was just wondering if there was any progress?'

'You know I can't speak about an ongoing investigation,' PC Shaw explained patiently.

'It's just that I'd heard it was a gang steaming and I was hoping you might have some information…'

'We are following all possible leads at this time.'

'I just thought I could maybe help with that – you know I saw the main guy briefly and I heard their voices,' I was desperate for her not to dismiss me like Damon and the others.

'If you want to come in and look at some photographs, that might be helpful to us.'

'Ok,' I agreed eagerly. We arranged a time and hung up.

When I turned up at Torphichen Street station PC Shaw was there to meet me. She ushered me into a back room where there were some folders on a table and three brown plastic chairs.

'It was only a brief glimpse,' I said, almost apologetic before we had even begun. The policewoman nodded understandingly.

'Just may jog a memory if you see him again,' she said quietly and opened the first of the folders.

I saw nothing in any of the motley assortment of faces which took me back to that day in the Carrier. Not in the first folder, nor in the second, but in the third there was a mugshot which made alarm bells begin to ring in my head. I pointed a shaking finger at the young man in the picture.

'He looks familiar,' I said, 'but I'm not sure. I only saw him briefly and he had a baseball cap on low. But it could have been this one…'

PC Shaw looked carefully at the photo I had indicated and nodded silently.

'Okay,' she said quietly. 'Thank you.'

'Is that it? What happens now? Do you go and arrest him?' I was desperate to find some finality.

'We'll keep you informed of any progress,' she replied cagily. 'Now the best thing you can do is go home and let us get on with things.'

Another dismissal. It rankled. But I smiled brightly and told her I hoped I'd been of some assistance and went to a nearby pub, wondering why the police hadn't shown me the photos before now.

8

Another week and still no word from PC Shaw. I called her again.

'Things are moving along. They just take time. We have to be certain,' she told me, sounding weary.

I tried calling Damon to suggest that he go and look at the photos too. After all, he'd had a much clearer view of the guy and, after much frustrated huffing, he agreed. PC Shaw did not sound pleased to hear from me again so soon but she assured me Damon would be called in.

I arranged to meet him in Carter's Bar after his visit to the station – it was just round the corner, and I went back to bed feeling a little more contented than I had for months.

9

Hamish had told stories of his days in the army, stationed in Malaya, Germany and Northern Ireland, leaving just before the Falklands War. He had been orphaned very young and brought up in an unemotional and abusive house by his aunt and uncle, leaving as soon as he was old enough to join up as a soldier. Witnessing countless comrades gunned down and blown up began to have an effect on him early on in his career and he had for some time been confined to doing office work at the barracks in Yorkshire, but his determination to see action again saw him back on the frontline within a couple of years. Sent to Northern Ireland at the height of the Troubles only served to compound his traumas and he ended his army days in a hospital being treated for a leg injury and PTSD. He would never lose either the limp or the night terrors.

Returning to Edinburgh after his discharge papers had been served, he found he had nowhere to go and knew no-one. He had booked into a hostel and taken to drinking through the day to make the nights less terrifying. There was no way he could hold down any kind of job and he became reliant on benefits and his army pension. Occasionally he would mention the names of his old friends lost in action and become tearful as he recalled their last moments, sometimes in his arms, but he would never talk of his own injury, simply limping a little more when the weather was cold or damp. Nor would he mention the abuse he suffered as a child except to say that this had heightened his post traumatic stress.

Damon and I, and probably countless others in a variety of pubs around the city, had heard these stories a hundred times in various forms until we were unsure as to which tales were true and which he was exaggerating. But, however one examined the situation, he had not deserved to die in the undignified manner he had and seemingly for no reason.

I lay alone in my bed once more and went over his stories in my head. 'That poor guy,' I thought. 'He had no luck in life or death.' Perhaps I should take stock of my own situation. I still had parents, grandparents and a brother with a wife and children. Friends of a sort. These were people who would miss me were I to become a crime statistic as Dirk had. And, if it was truly as random as it seemed to be, who was to say it wouldn't be me next? I resolved to call my whole family the next day.

10

My guilt assuaged as far as my family went, I continued my hounding of PC Shaw, despite the fact that she would never tell me anything until, one day, four months after Dirk's death, she called to tell me they had arrested the guy both Damon and I had identified and charged him with aggravated murder. They had not caught, nor had he given up, any of the rest of the gang from that day, but it was progress, they assured me. I felt a huge surge of relief and telephoned Damon to let him know.

'See, and you said I'd lose it,' I said with a tone of triumph.

'You did a bit,' he replied, but I could hear the smile in his voice.